BY ANN DUGAN AND
THE EDITORS OF CONSUMER GUIDE®

*NEW PROGRAM:*
*1 INCH OFF IN ONE WEEK*

# FLATTEN YOUR STOMACH

## FOR WORKING WOMEN

BEEKMAN HOUSE
New York

Louis Weber, President
Publications International, Ltd.
3841 West Oakton Street
Skokie, Illinois 60076

Permission is never granted for commercial purposes.

Printed and bound in Yugoslavia by CGP Delo
10  9  8  7  6  5  4  3  2  1

Library of Congress Catalog Card Number: 86-60769

ISBN: 0-517-61677-7

Design: Inez Smith
Photography: Sam Griffith Studios
Model: Dale Fahey

This edition published by
Beekman House
Distributed by Crown Publishers, Inc.

# CONTENTS

# THE 7 DAY PROGRAM

No time to work out? No energy left at the end of the day? You still have that midriff bulge, belt overhang, and a stomach you can't even pull in any more? The all new **Flatten Your Stomach for Working Women** program is the exercise plan for you.

Everyone wants a flat stomach. We all want the attractive, fit, youthful look of a narrow waist, a firm abdomen. Of course, paying attention to what you eat is essential to your health and fitness. But weight loss alone will not give you the firm, flat stomach you want. What really gives a body a terrific shape is well-toned muscles.

Think of it this way: the muscles that allow you to perform your daily tasks on the job and at home are also the muscles that give you your shape. If they are well toned, strong, firm, and resilient, you will have a good figure. However, there are few daily activities that sufficiently exercise the abdominal muscles. Even gravity seems to fight you in your efforts to achieve or maintain a slender, trim shape.

Proper exercise can shape up any stomach, no matter how far gone. But you need a regular, carefully planned exercise program. You need a program that tones all the muscles in the abdomen. There are four major abdominal muscles. Some of these muscles run up and down. Others run side to side. Some crisscross the abdomen at an angle. If you exercise only one of these muscles (say, by doing only sit-ups), your stomach may be hard, but it won't be flat.

The **Flatten Your Stomach** program is based on the latest research in the fields of Sports Medicine, Kinesiology, and Physiology. Just a few exercises each day will start you on the path to getting the flat stomach, trim waistline, slender figture you want—and help you keep it that way!

The **Flatten Your Stomach for Working Women** program recognizes that you have little time to devote to yourself, but you want to look good and be healthy. It gives you an exercise plan for every day of the week. Each exercise routine takes only about 30 minutes. The exercises are foolproof and easy to follow. The entire program has been designed to produce balanced muscle development and shaping, while avoiding injury and soreness. Follow this simple program, exercising regularly and vigorously each day. You'll feel more fit, energetic, self-confident, and attractive in no time.

The **Flatten Your Stomach for Working Women** program is different from other exercise plans you may have tried. It is designed just for YOU—the working woman. For any exercise plan to be useful, you have to follow it. The 7 Day Program is flexible; it allows you to fit some of your exercises into your busy working schedule. You use your daily activities (such as walking up and down stairs, running for the train, walking, even housework) as a springboard; you are then ready to jump into the rest of your workout—at a time that's convenient for YOU.

## FOLLOWING THE PROGRAM

**The Flatten Your Stomach for Working Women** program begins with warm-ups, which prepare your body for exercise. A series of stretches help condition the back. Now you move into the main section of the program—focusing your attention and concentrating your efforts on those exercises designed specifically to flatten and tighten the muscles of the abdominal region. A cool-down period helps your body return to its pre-exercise state—leaving you invigorated, relaxed, and feeling really good about yourself.

The program offers seven new exercise routines—a new routine for every day of the week. The exercises gradually progress from Day 1 on, so that Days 6 and 7, for example, are more difficult than Days 1 and 2. You may sometimes want to arrange your exercise program so that you do the routines for Day 1 or 2 when you may have less time or energy to devote to exercise.

*Warm-ups* get your body going. They generally loosen up the muscles all over your body and get your heart and lungs working at higher levels. Warm-ups are essential for two main reasons.

When your body is properly warmed up, the more vigorous stomach exercises will be more effective. Warm-ups raise the body and muscle temperature to efficient levels. They increase the blood supply in the muscles and increase the rate and force of muscle contractions. Your car works more efficiently after the engine is properly warmed up. The same is true for your body.

Warm-ups also make you less prone to injury when you move on to more vigorous exercises. They stretch the ligaments and tissues to permit greater flexibility. By gradually activating muscle fibers, you'll help prevent muscle tears and strains. How will you know when you've warmed up enough? You'll be slightly out of breath, and you'll break the "sweat barrier."

The exercises for the stomach are a combination of spot exercises and stretches. Our *spot exercises* are muscle-toners, not "spot reducers." Exercising one area of the body will not reduce the amount of fat in that area. However, our spot exercises can change the shape of an area. Restoring muscle tone makes the abdomen firmer and more attractively shaped.

*Stretches* are also included with each day's exercise routine. Stretches help you avoid injury by increasing flexibility and range of movement. The connective tissues of your body are like rubber bands. If not stretched frequently, the tissues become tight and limit your movement. If not stretched at all for a long time, the tissues may snap, causing injury and pain. Take the stretches slowly at first. Do not stretch any farther than you feel comfortable. As the ligaments gradually loosen, your stretches will go farther.

The *stomach-flattening* exercises are carefully designed to help your muscles develop evenly. This even development of all the abdomen's different muscles is what gives you the shape and proportion you're after. Our exercise routines carefully alternate the muscles exercised. One exercise may work on the muscles that run up and down the abdomen. The next may firm up those that run side to side. Another may work on the muscles that crisscross the abdomen. That is one good reason to do all the exercises in each routine in the order given.

*Cool downs* are exercises that allow your body to slow down gradually. After strenuous work, the body must readjust to pre-exercise levels of body function. Cool downs help your muscles begin to relax. They allow your circulatory system to slow down gradually. If you stop exercising suddenly, without this tapering-off period, blood collects in the muscles and veins. This could cause dizziness and weakness. A proper cool down also helps mimimize soreness and stiffness.

The term *"sets"* in the **Flatten Your Stomach for Working Women** program refers to the number of times you should repeat a group of exercises before stopping (for example, "Repeat 8 times"). After the listed number of repetitions it is recommended that you rest briefly before beginning again. Resting between sets of repetitions allows muscles to restore their energy reserves, so that they are ready to continue contracting without injury or cramping. As you progress on the 7 Day Program you might want to add more sets. However, always remember to rest between sets.

# THE 7 DAY PROGRAM

The length of time you need to rest depends largely upon your own conditioning. It is generally recommended that you rest long enough for your breathing to return to normal. When you start the program, you may need to rest for as long as one to two minutes between sets. But as your endurance improves, your rest periods should become shorter.

Unless a specific breathing pattern is indicated, try to *breathe* normally through your mouth and nose. Never take deep breaths, and never hold your breath.

Notice that some of the exercises recommend a particular breathing procedure. Exhale as you do the exercise, inhale as you relax. Thus you exhale as your abdominal muscles contract and are under stress, inhale when they are under the least amount of stress.

## MAKING IT WORK

To the get most from the time and energy you put into this program, keep these guidelines in mind.

● Wear comfortable clothing that allows you to move freely, such as shorts, a leotard, or a light exercise suit.

● Exercise in tennis shoes, in socks, or barefoot—whatever is most comfortable to you. If you have a weak back, weak knees, or weak ankles, wear tennis shoes or running shoes.

● If possible, exercise on a wooden floor or on a carpet. Exercising on concrete surfaces can be hard on your body. For floor exercises, try to work on a mat, a carpet remnant, a piece of foam rubber, or a folded towel.

● Try to exercise every day, or at least four times a week. A regular exercise program offers the most benefit for your body.

● Establish your own exercise schedule. You shouldn't exercise just before bedtime or just after you eat. Most any other time is fine. Once you choose the best time, stick to it. Exercising at the same time every day helps you develop the exercise habit.

● Follow the routines carefully. If you follow directions, you should tone and shape muscles properly, avoid injury, and suffer a minimum of soreness.

● If you cannot do an exercise exactly as it is described, don't worry. Try it, and then go on to the next exercise. Don't feel discouraged. As you increase your strength and flexibility, you will eventually be able to do most of the exercises. Then you will realize just how far you have progressed.

● Remember that your individual body structure may make an exercise difficult for you. Body structure and flexibility vary greatly from person to person. The structure of your joints or the length of your arms or legs may prevent you from doing an exercise exactly as it is described. Don't push yourself past your own body's limits. Aim toward what is asked for in each exercise, doing the best that you can.

● Do the number of repetitions given in the text, until the exercises are easy for you. Then gradually increase the number of repetitions for each exercise. For some exercises, the text recommends the number of repetitions you should try to work toward. In general, you might aim toward eventually doubling the repetitions given in the text. But don't try to go too far too fast. Add only a few at a time.

● At the end of each day's exercises, you should feel a healthy, relaxed sense of fatigue. Exercise that does not tax the body does not help the body.

● No matter how rushed you may be, do not neglect to do the warm-ups and cool downs. These exercises are essential for keeping your body flexible, getting your heart and lungs working efficiently, and avoiding injury and stiffness.

● As you work through each day's routine, keep your body moving. You lose some of the benefits if you take long breaks between exercises. Exercising to lively music can help you pace yourself and really keep you going. However, it is important to rest briefly between "sets."

● Learn to listen to your body for signs of fatigue. You want to exercise vigorously enough to work up a sweat. But be careful not to overdo. If you're winded and breathless, or if you suffer sprains or stitches in the side, assume that you're exercising too vigorously. Slow down a little.

● If you haven't exercised for a while, it is normal to be a little sore and stiff when you first start. Stiffness does not mean you should stop moving. In most cases, it means you should get going again. Remember that warming up and cooling down properly will help minimize soreness.

● If you think you may be injured, stop using the injured limb. Continuing to exercise could worsen the injury. Stop your exercise program until the injury no longer hurts when you are at rest. Then gradually begin to exercise slowly and carefully.

● To avoid back problems, always to sit-ups with the knees bent. When lifting your back off the floor or lowering your back to the floor, keep your head up, chin toward the chest. Curl the back as you lift and lower it. Also curl your back when you bend the torso over and return to an upright position.

● If you feel any tightness or discomfort in your back, take a break for a few minutes. The abdominal muscles depend on the back for much of their support. Therefore, some exercises for the abdomen may also put some strain on the back. This is especially true if your back is weak. These exercises will gradually help strengthen the back, but go slowly at first.

● If you have weak ankles or weak knees, be careful during exercises that put stress on the ankles or knees. Take it easy until you start to strengthen the muscles in those areas.

● Supplement this program with as much activity as possible. You should consciously aim at becoming a more physically active person. Try to do more walking, bicycling, dancing. Take the stairs instead of the elevator. Participate in whatever active sports you enjoy. Keep that energy level up.

● Don't be discouraged if you gain a little weight after the first week of exercise. A small weight gain means that the muscles are becoming firmer and denser. Those few extra pounds will disappear after another week of regular exercise.

● If you miss a week or more on this program, start again with the number of repetitions given in the text. You'll have to rebuild your strength and flexibility before increasing the number of repetitions again.

● All the exercises in this program were developed in consultation with medical experts. However, it is recommended that you consult your doctor before beginning this or any program of exercise.

## ON YOUR WAY

Now let's get started. You have the ground rules. You understand how this terrific program works. So get into some comfortable clothes, put on some upbeat music, and get moving. It will take some effort, but it will all be worth it. Don't expect overnight results. But you'll soon notice that you're looking a little bit better every day you exercise. Within only a few weeks, this program can shape you up dramatically. The **Flatten Your Stomach** program will take only a few minutes each day, but the rewards can last a lifetime. Much sooner than you think, you can shape up, slim down, and look terrific!

# POWER
# SWITCH ON
## WARM UP

**1**

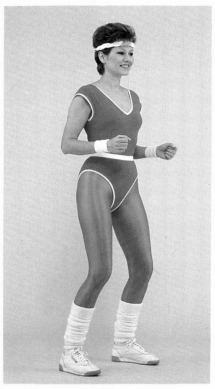

Stand with your feet slightly apart, knees bent. Bend your arms at waist height, ready for action.

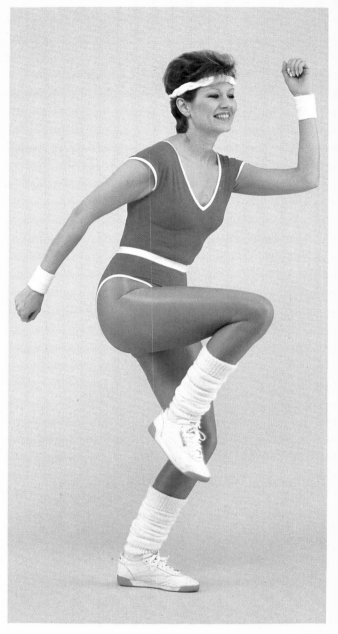

**2** Run for a few minutes, or until you feel "unwound" and ready to exercise.

*This run is to loosen you up and "rev up" your energy level.*

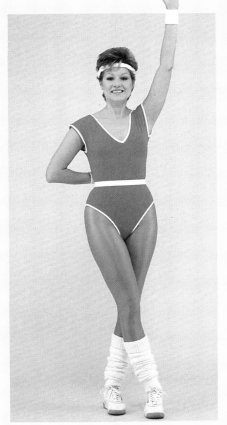

**1**

Stand with your weight on your left foot, and cross your right foot in front of the left. Bend your right arm behind your back, and extend your left arm upward.

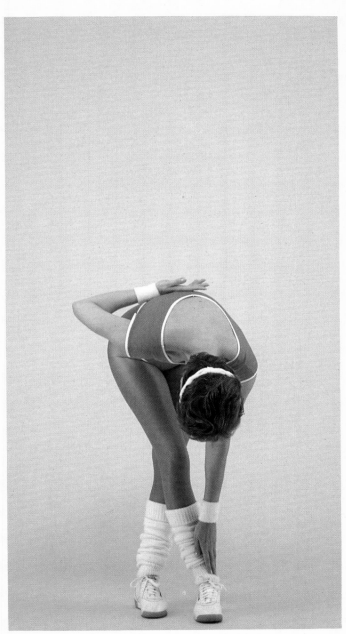

**2** S-l-o-w-l-y bend over, sliding the left hand down the right leg toward your ankle. Hold for 5 counts. Return to position 1, then repeat, using the right arm and left leg.

# PULL UP

## Warm Up

**1**

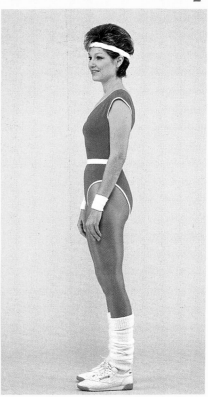

Stand erect, with your feet slightly apart, your arms relaxed at your sides.

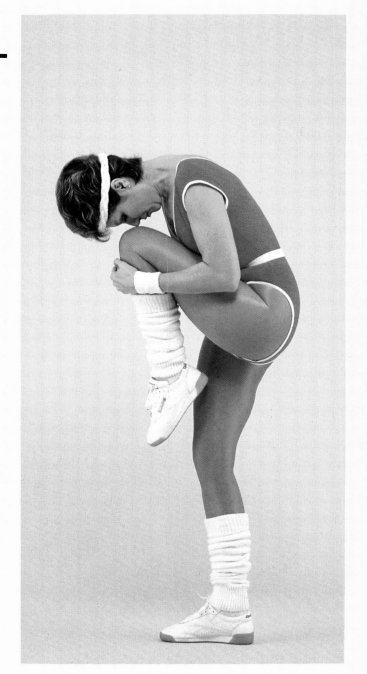

**2** Grasp your left knee with both hands and pull it up toward your chest. Touch your nose to your knee. Try to hold for 5 counts. Return to position 1, then repeat with the right knee. Alternate left and right knees, 3 times each.

*This exercise is used to relieve tension, and to stretch the tight ligaments in the back.*

# *1*

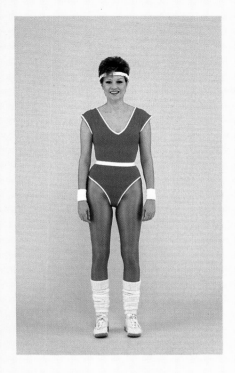

Stand with your feet together, arms at your sides.

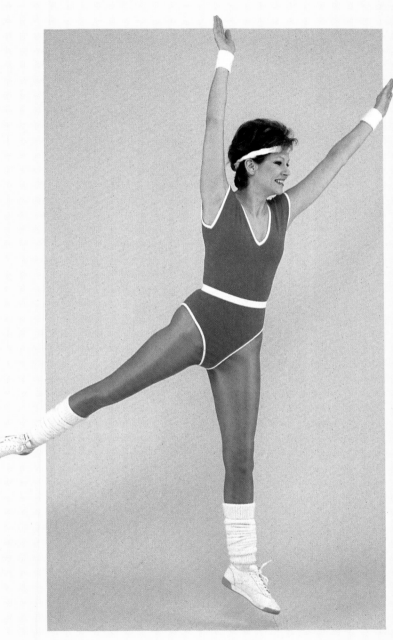

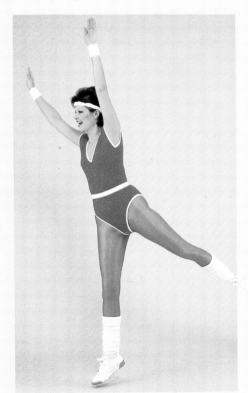

*2* Hop on your right foot, extending your left leg behind you. Swing both arms upward to the right.

*3* Repeat, bouncing on your left foot and swinging your arms upward to the left. Continue, alternating right and left for two sets of 8 swings each.

*Do this exercise in a swinging, dance-step movement.*

# SIMPLE BUT STRONG

## *Warm Up*

**1**

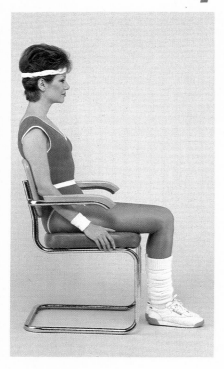

Sit erect in a stable, straight chair, with your back flat against the back of the chair. Place your feet flat on the floor and grasp the seat of the chair.

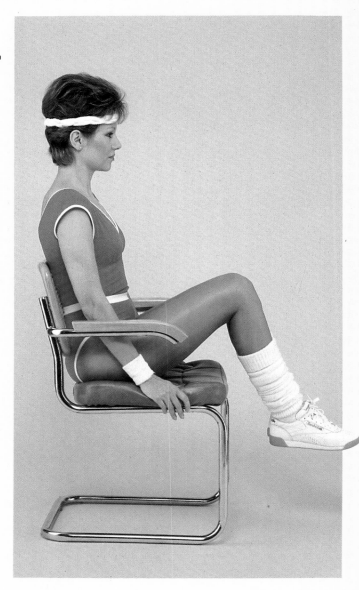

**2** Lift both feet off of the floor, raising your knees as high as possible. Lower your legs to the floor. Repeat for 3 sets of 8 bends.

*A simple, but very effective exercise that you can do anywhere, anytime, as often as possible during the day.*

**1**

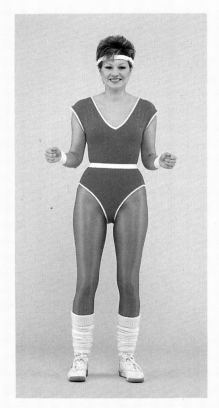

Stand with your feet together, knees slightly bent. Arms are bent, and held at waist level.

# THE TWIST

*Warm Up*

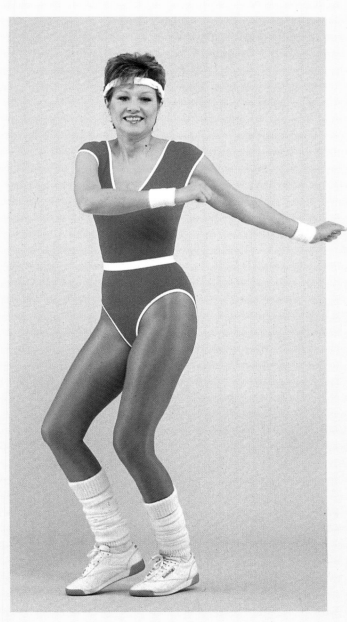

**2** Slide on the balls of your feet, turning your toes to the right, hips to the left. Swing your arms to the left. Put on some upbeat music and alternate twisting left and right for the length of a song (approximately 3 minutes).

# TIGHT SQUEEZE

## DAY 1

**1**

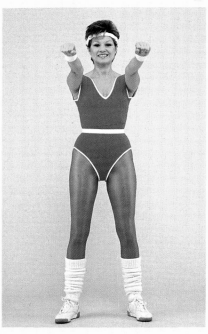

Stand with your feet wide apart, arms extended straight forward, hands held in fists. Face forward; avoid twisting your head.

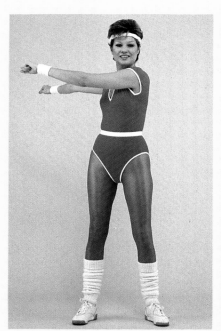

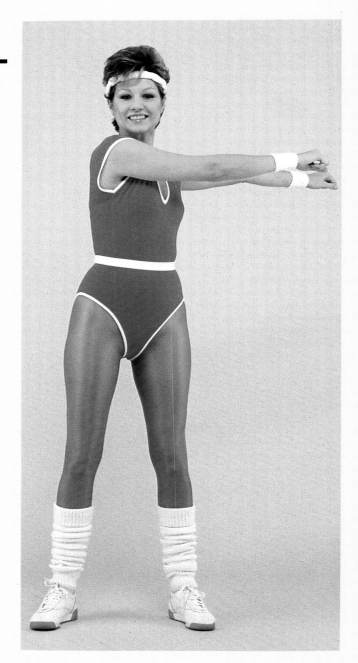

**3** Move them to the left (4 times left, 4 times right). Drop your arms, rest, then repeat. Rest, then continue—for a total of 24 swings in each direction.

**2** Keeping your arms straight, vigorously move them to the right, across your chest.

**1**

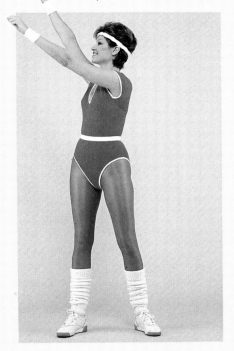

Stand with legs far apart, arms at your sides, hands held in fists.

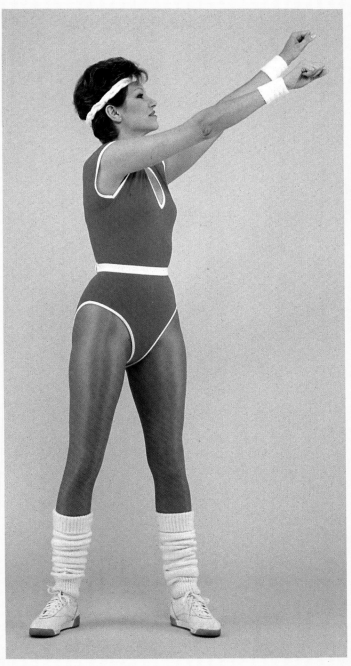

**2**

Keeping your arms straight, move both arms upward and across to the right. At the same time turn your upper torso and head to the right, so that your eyes follow your hands.

**3** Return to position 1, then swing your arms upward to the left. Repeat, alternating right and left for a total of 8 swings. Rest, then repeat 2 more sets of 8 swings.

# TURN IN

*Day 1*

**1**

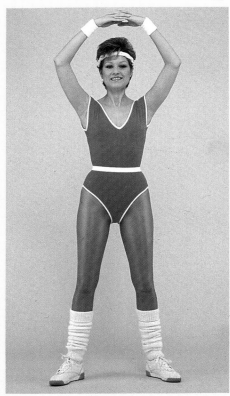

Face forward. Stand with your feet wide apart, arms extended upward, elbows slightly bent, hands clasped overhead.

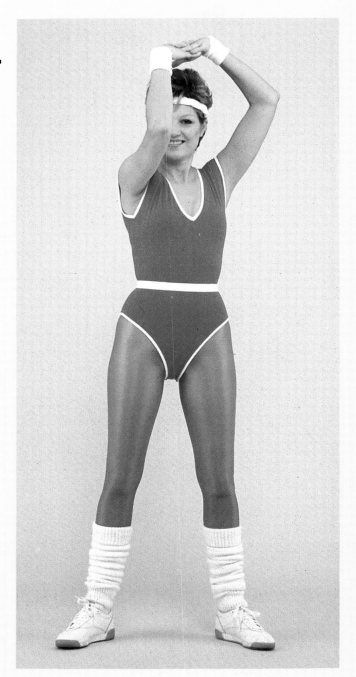

**2** Maintaining the upper torso position, pull your right elbow in toward the center of your body until it is directly in front of your eyes. Return to position 1. Repeat 8 times, then repeat using your left elbow. Rest, then repeat for a total of 3 sets of 8 pulls on each side.

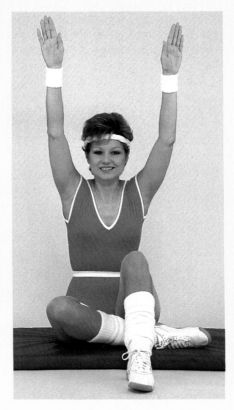

Sit on the floor with your left knee bent up so that the left foot rests on the floor; your right ankle rests on the floor below your left knee. Hold your arms straight up above your head.

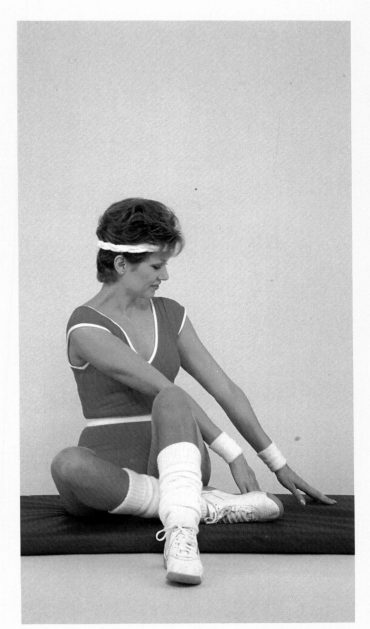

**2** Very s-l-o-w-l-y lower both arms, passing outside the left knee toward the floor at the left hip. At the same time, turn the upper torso and follow your arms with your eyes. Move smoothly, without any jerking motions. Hold for 5 counts. Return to position 1 and repeat on the right side. Repeat for a total of 8 times on each side.

# SIDE SWEEP

## Day 1

*You should feel a pinch at the waist and a strong pull and tightening of the lower abdominal muscle group.*

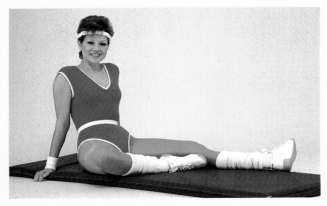

**1** Sit on the floor with your right knee bent outward, left leg extended straight forward. Use your hands to support your body at the hips.

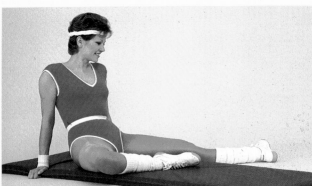

**2** Slowly move your left leg to the left side as far as possible.

**3** Try to trace out a boxlike pattern with your left foot—out, up, in, and down. Return to position 1. Repeat 8 times. Repeat, shifting position, and moving the right leg to the right. Repeat for a total of 3 sets of 8 sweeps on each side.

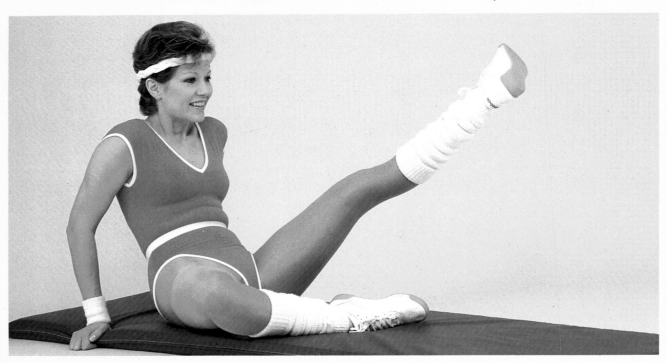

**1**

Sit on the floor with your left leg bent upward, left foot on the floor, right knee bent outward. The sole of your right foot should rest against the instep of your left foot. Bend the elbows and grasp the knees for support.

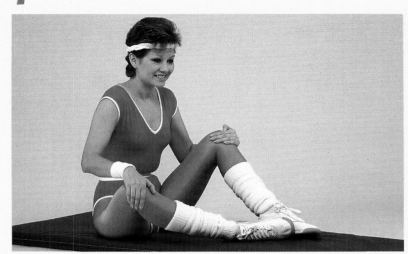

**2** S-l-o-w-l-y press the upper torso backward, until your arms are straight. Hold. Return to position 1. Repeat for a total of 24 times (resting between each group of 8). Switch sides and repeat (24 times).

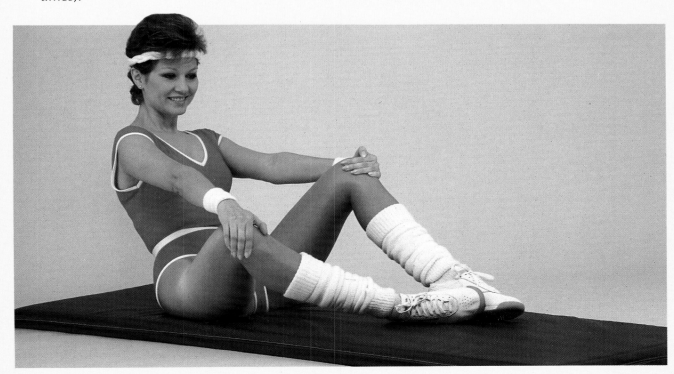

# WHITTLE THE MIDDLE

*This exercise is essential. It helps stretch and provide flexibility of the back, so that the back will be strong enough to support abdominal exercises without injury.*

## Day 1

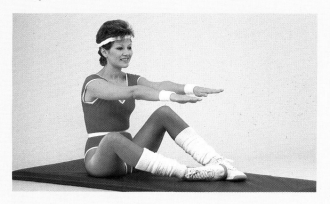

**1** Sit on the floor with the left knee bent upward, right knee bent outward, left foot flat on the floor. Extend your arms horizontally in front of you.

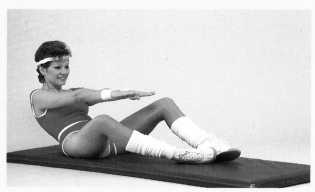

**2** Keeping the back rounded, lean back until contraction is felt in the muscles of your lower abdomen. Hold 5 counts.

**3** Swing forward, straighten the left leg, and touch your left ankle with both hands. Return to position 1 and repeat 8 times. Reverse leg positions and repeat 8 times. Continue, for a total of 4 sets of 8 times each, alternating left and right sides.

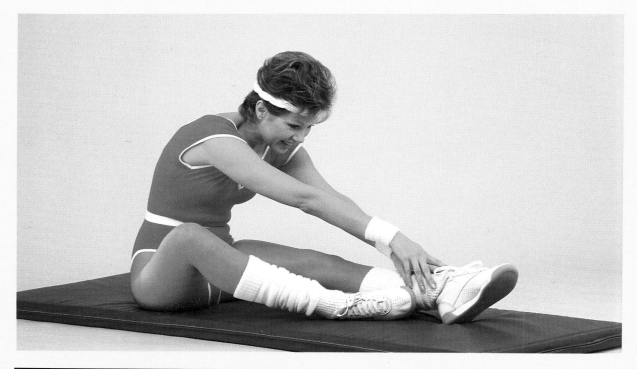

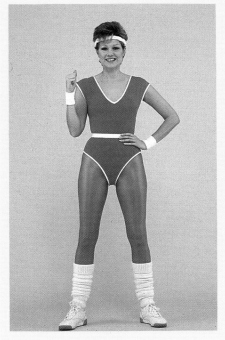

# 1     PUNCH OUT

## DAY 2

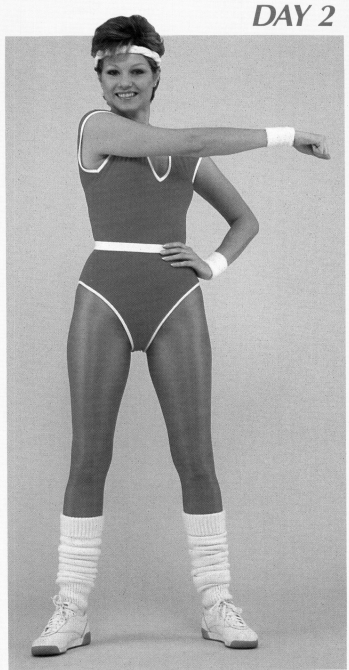

Stand with your feet wide apart, left hand on your hip. Bend your right arm, holding your hand in a fist at shoulder level. Keep your head and eyes forward—do not twist.

## 2

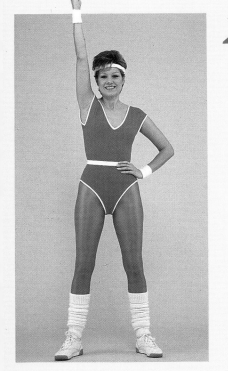

Thrust the right arm straight up overhead, then return to position 1.

**3**   Strongly thrust the right arm across the body, extending it to the left side. Return to position 1 and repeat steps 2 and 3, 8 times. Reverse arm positions and repeat 8 times. Continue, for a total of 2 sets on each side.

*This exercise is super for "rolls" around the middle—put a lot of muscle into this one.*

# FEEL LEAN

## Day 2

**1**

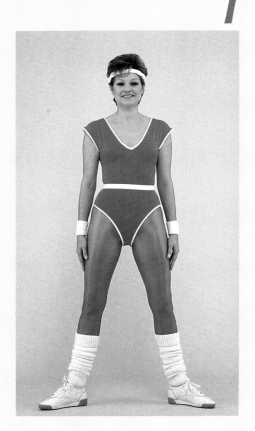

Stand erect, with your feet wide apart, toes turned out slightly, arms held at your sides.

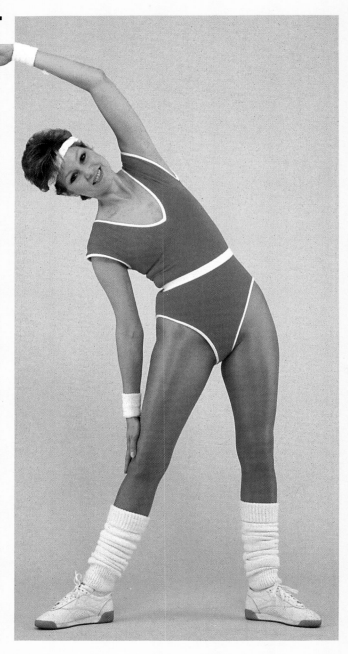

**2** S-l-o-w-l-y bend toward the right as far as possible, sliding the right hand down the right leg. At the same time, raise the left arm and arch it overhead and to the right in a long stretch. Return to position 1 and repeat, alternating left and right for a total of 16 stretches.

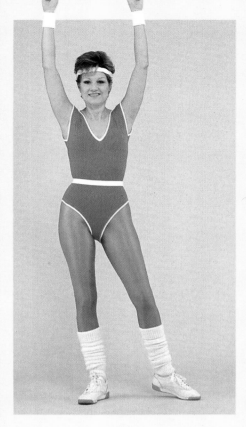

Stand with your feet slightly apart, weight on the right foot, left knee slightly bent. Arms are extended straight overhead, with hands held in fists.

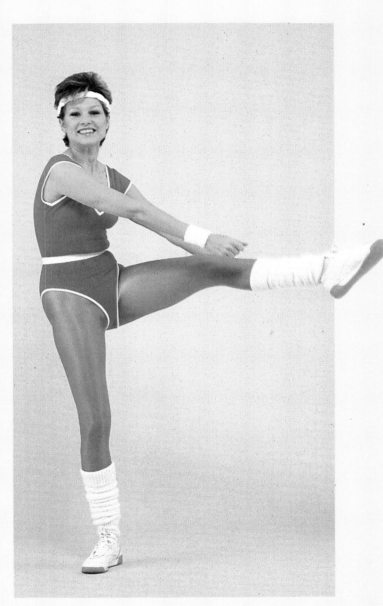

**2** Raise your left leg directly to the side. At the same time, lower both arms downward and to the left, keeping your elbows as straight as possible. Do not twist or turn your body sideways toward the left leg. Lower the left leg and return to position 1. Repeat, this time raising the right leg. Continue for a total of 16 times, alternating right and left sides.

# DELETE
# THE WAIST

## Day 2

**1**

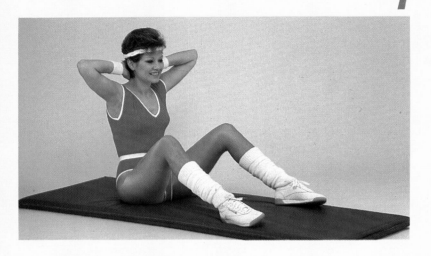

Sit on the floor. Bend the knees and place your feet flat on the floor and wide apart. Clasp your hands behind your head, with the elbows spread.

*This exercise causes strong contraction of the lateral oblique muscles at the sides of the waist—for a "Scarlet O'Hara waistline."*

Twist to the right and place your left elbow outside your right knee. Return to position 1. Twist to the left, and place your right elbow outside your left knee. Repeat, for a total of 16 twists, alternating left and right. Do this exercise smoothly—do not jerk forcefully or twist your head.

**2**

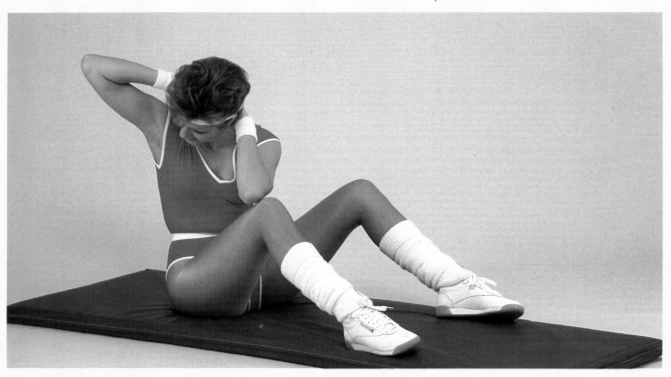

**1**

Sit on the floor with your knees bent, back erect. Hold your arms at your sides, with the elbows bent. Grasp the back of your thighs.

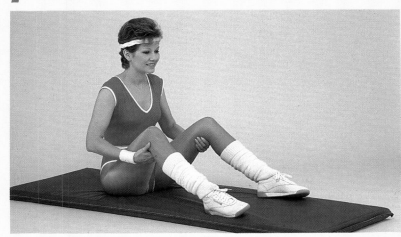

Keeping your head and shoulders forward, curl your chest and torso, so that your pelvis is tilted upward. Lean back until your arms are straight (exhale as you lean back). Hold position for 5 seconds. Return to position 1 (inhale as you sit up). Repeat for 2 sets of 8 times each.

*This is one of several exercises that are designed strictly for the area of the lower abdomen (belly).*

**2**

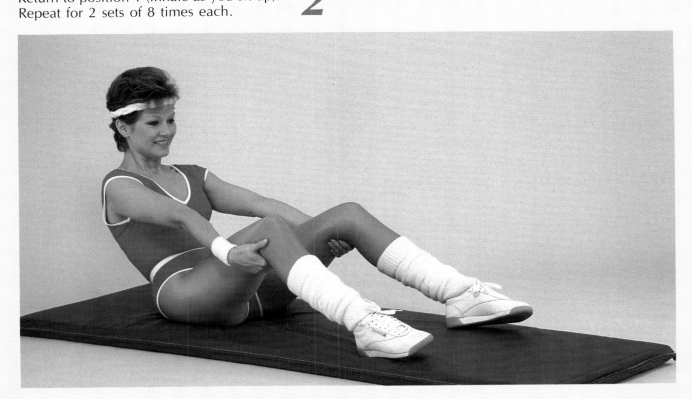

# BATTLE
# THE BULGE

*Day 2*

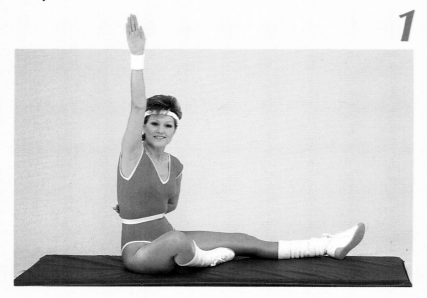

**1**

Sit on the floor with your left leg extended to the left, toe pointed upward, the right knee bent outward. Fold your left arm behind your back and extend your right arm upward.

*You should feel a pinching at the waistline as you stretch.*

**2** Bending to the left in a long stretch, touch your right hand to your left toe. Return to position 1 and repeat 8 times. Switch sides and repeat 8 times on the right. Continue for a total of 2 sets on each side.

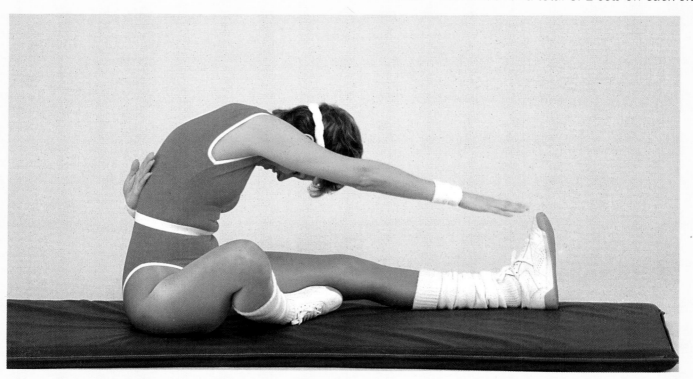

**1**

Lie with your head and feet resting on the floor, knees bent, legs wide apart. Clasp your hands behind your head at the base of the skull.

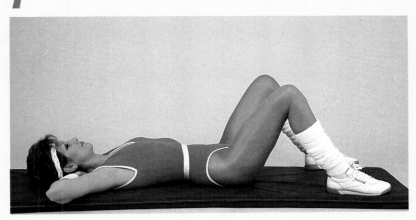

S-l-o-w-l-y lift your head and pull your elbows forward. Curl your head and shoulders upward until the small of the back is pushed into the floor. At the same time tilt your pelvis upward (exhale as you sit up). Hold the position for 5 counts. Return to position 1 and repeat 8 times.

*Do this exercise slowly—do not jerk your head or lift your shoulders too high. This exercise helps to tighten the lower abdominal muscles and strengthen the back.*

**2**

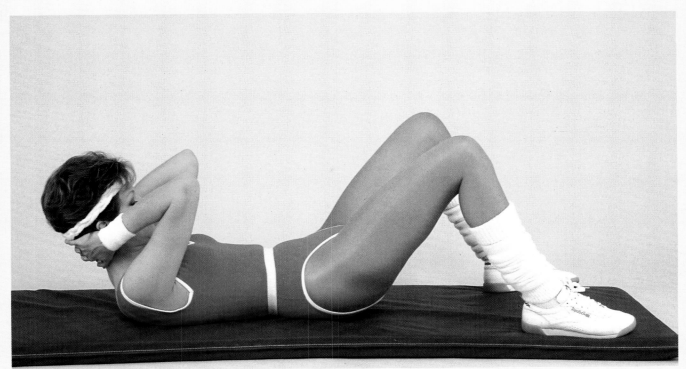

# SQUEEZE UP

## DAY 3

**1**

Standing erect with your weight on the right foot, arms overhead, point your left leg behind you, with weight on the toe. Look upward, and arch your back slightly in a long stretch.

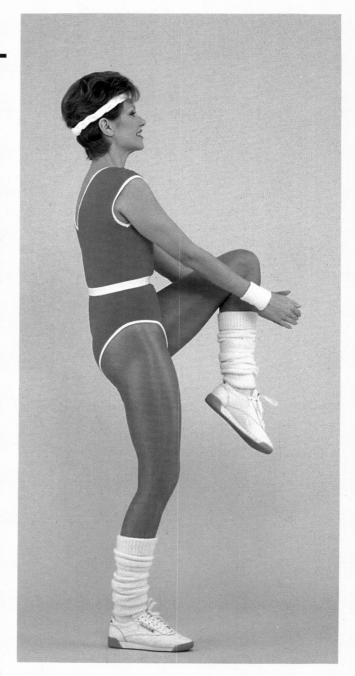

**2** Raise your left knee upward, toward the chest. At the same time, lower both arms to encircle the knee. Compress the abdomen by hugging the knee closely to the chest. Return to position 1, making sure your left leg is extended straight backward. Repeat 8 times left; 8 times right. Continue for a total of 2 sets on each side.

*This exercise not only firms the abdominal muscles, but also helps to eliminate cramping and bloating.*

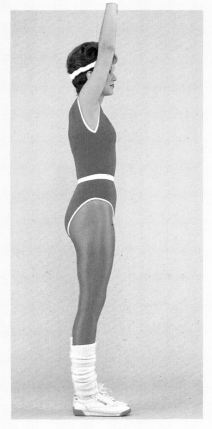

**1**

Stand erect with your feet together, arms extended overhead.

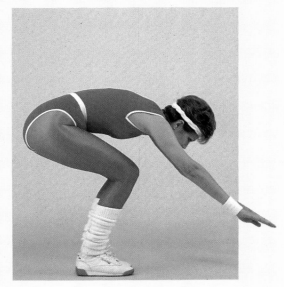

**2**

Bend your knees and swing your arms downward, lowering the torso to the knees.

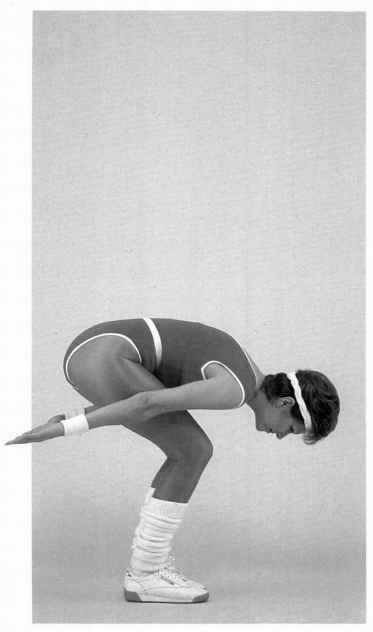

**3** Bounce once with your thighs parallel to the floor. (Do not jerk your head!) Follow through with your arms, swinging them upward behind you (in a skiing motion). Bounce once and return to position 1. Repeat 8 times.

*This exercise helps alleviate bloating.*

# TIGHTEN THE TUMMY

**Day 3**

**1**

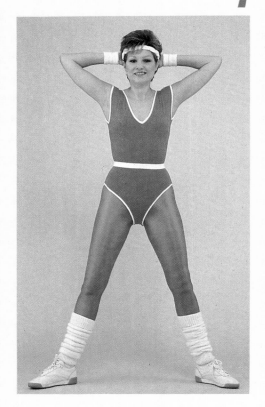

Stand erect with your feet wide apart, toes turned outward. Clasp your hands behind your head with the elbows wide apart. Hold your head slightly forward.

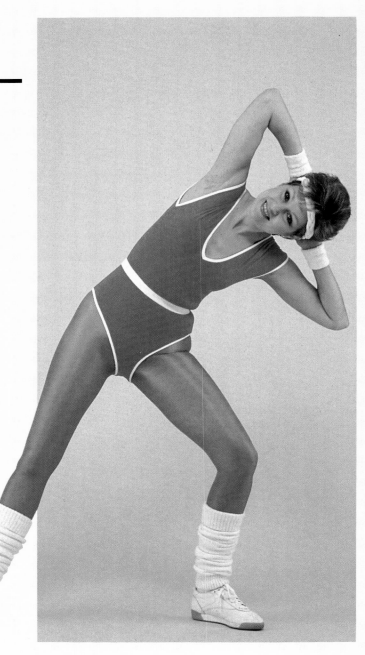

**2** Bend your left knee outward. Lean to the left and incline your left elbow toward your left knee. (Do not twist your body; keep it erect and *lean* sideways.) Smoothly return to position 1 and repeat, using your right elbow and right knee. Repeat for 3 sets of 8 bends each, alternating left and right.

*This is a great exercise for "belt overhang"—it helps firm the waist, hips, and thighs.*

*This exercise not only firms the abdomen, but strengthens the back as well.*

# LONG RANGE RESULTS
## Day 3

**1** Sit with your knees bent, feet flat on the floor. Fold your arms across your chest.

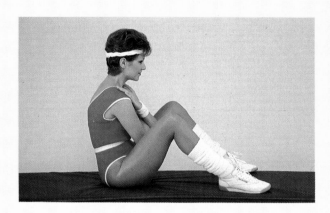

**2** Keeping your head and shoulders forward and arms across your chest, slowly lean back with your body curled slightly. Lean back until the back of your pelvis tilts upward (or as far as you are able to lean). Hold for 5 counts. Exhale.

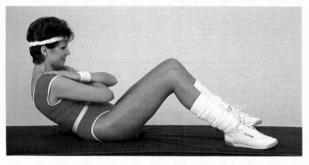

**3** Return to position 1, then reach forward between your legs with both hands as far as possible (inhale as you move). Repeat full cycle for 3 sets of 8 times each.

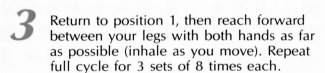

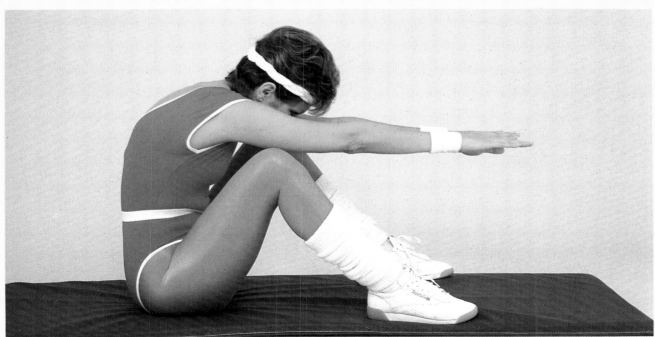

# OVER EASY

*Day 3*

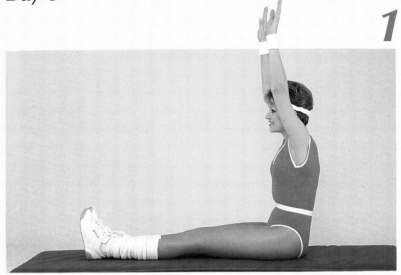

**1**

Sit with the legs together and extended straight forward, toes up. Extend the arms straight overhead.

*This is a terrific exercise for the central abdomen. It also helps firm the hamstring muscles at the back of the legs.*

Bend the knees slightly and at the same time lean forward and touch your toes with both hands. Reach forward just as far as you possibly can. Return to position 1 and repeat, for 3 sets of 8 times each.

**2**

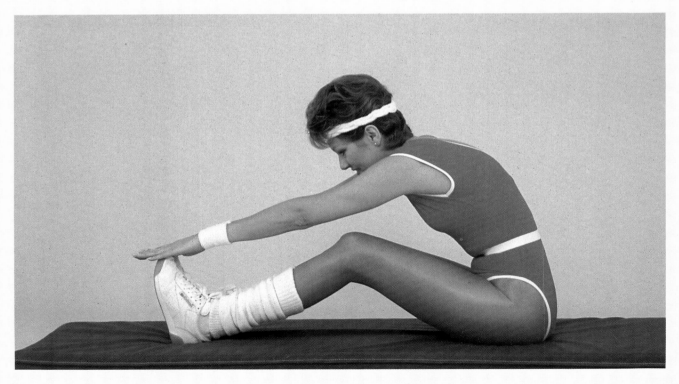

**1**

Sit with your body erect, legs wide apart, hands on the floor at your sides.

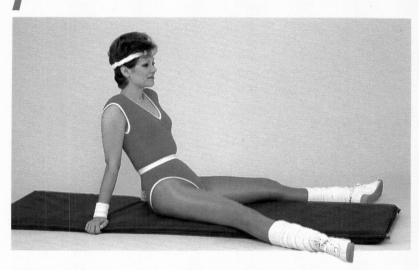

**2** Put your weight on your right hand and swing your left arm across your body, upward and to the left. At the same time, rolling on your right hip, raise your left leg, lifting it as high as possible. Return to position 1, then repeat 8 times left, 8 times right. Continue for 3 sets of 8 each, alternating left and right.

*This is a complete abdominal exercise that uses all of the muscles of the abdomen. Do it in a very fluid, dance-like movement.*

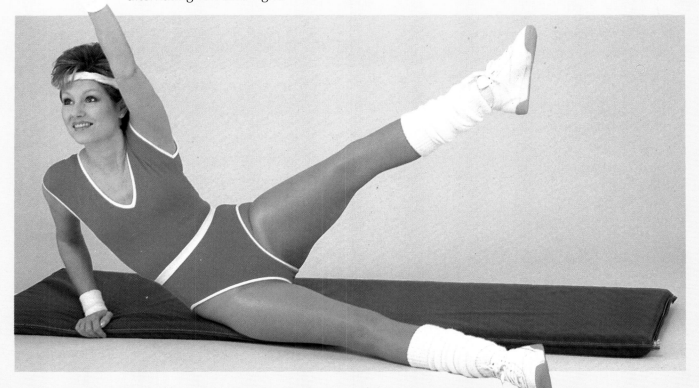

# STRONG INPUT

## Day 3

**1**

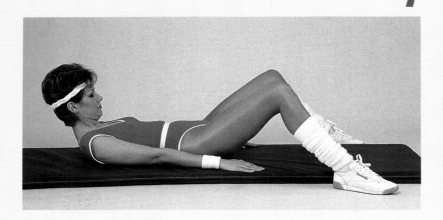

Lie on your back with your legs wide apart, knees bent, feet flat on the floor. Rest your hands on the floor at your sides. Lift your head up off the floor, chin on your chest.

Lift your head and shoulders slightly off the ground. At the same time, slide your hands and arms forward until you feel a strong contraction of the abdominal muscles. Exhale, and hold this position for 3 counts. Inhale as you return to position 1. Repeat 8 times. Repeat for a total of 3 sets of 8 lifts each, resting your head on the floor between sets.

*This is a very strong abdominal exercise that also helps strengthen the back.*

**2**

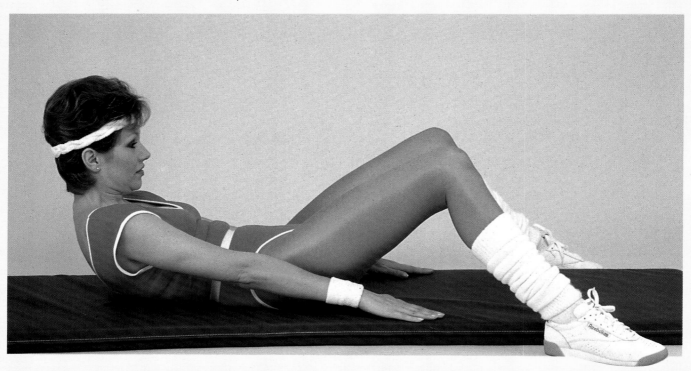

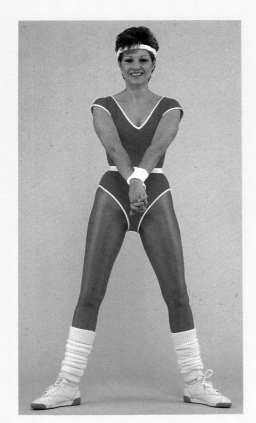

*1* Stand with your feet wide apart, knees slightly bent, toes pointed slightly to the sides. Arms are crossed in front of the body with the hands clasped. It is important that your arms remain straight—almost stiff.

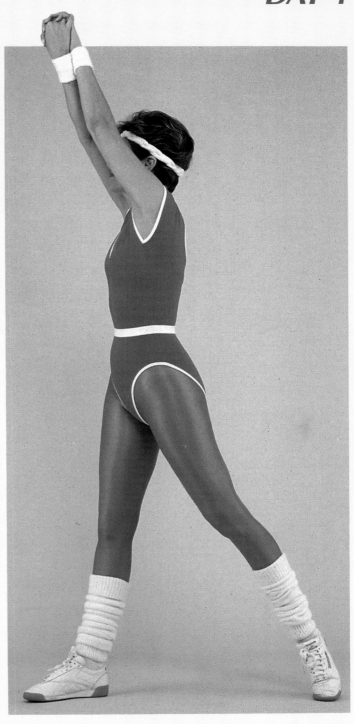

*2* Swing your arms upward to the right. At the same time, turn to the right side with your weight on the right foot; pivot on the left toe. Return to position 1. Swing to the left, shifting your weight onto your left foot. Repeat, alternating left and right for 8 swings. Continue for 3 sets of 8 each.

*If you do this exercise correctly you should feel the pull from the waistline to the shoulders.*

# SUBTRACT THE INCHES

**Day 4**

1

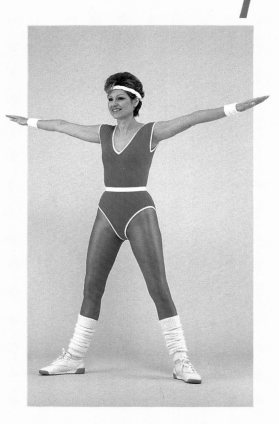

Stand with your feet wide apart, toes turned to the side. Arms are extended straight to the sides.

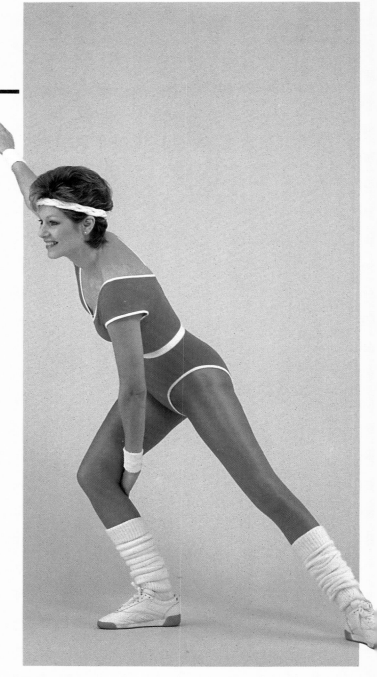

2 Bend the right knee and place your left hand behind it (use a swinging motion on the bend). At the same time, swing your right arm high behind you. Return to position 1. Repeat 8 times right, 8 times left. Continue for a total of 3 sets of 8 each.

*This exercise helps get rid of "bikini bulge." Do it in a fluid, waltz-type beat. Do not jerk your head.*

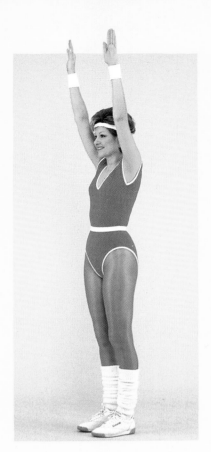

**1**

Stand with your feet together, arms extended straight overhead.

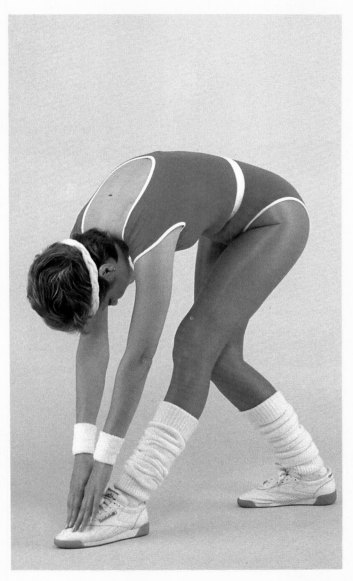

*This is a ballet movement; do it smoothly. It contracts and tones three abdominal muscle groups—this makes it a good all-around stomach firmer.*

**2** Bend your right knee and step forward with the left foot, keeping the left knee straight and toe pointed. Bend from the waist, lowering your arms at the same time. Touch your ankle. Return to position 1 and repeat 3 more times. Switch sides and repeat 4 times. Continue for 3 sets of 8, alternating right and left every 4 bends.

# PROJECT TIGHT MUSCLES

## Day 4

*These are strong exercises—if you feel a pull in your back, do them while resting on your elbows.*

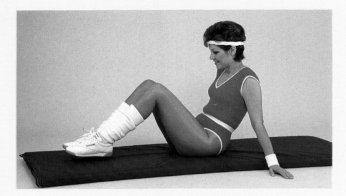

**1** Sit with your legs together, knees bent to the chest, feet barely off of the floor, hands supporting your body at the hips. Round your back and hunch your shoulders slightly to support the back.

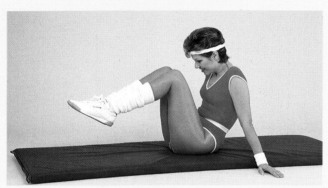

**2** Lift your knees toward your chest. Hold for 5 counts. Return to position 1 and repeat 8 times. Continue for 3 sets of 8 each.

**3** Lift your knees toward your chest. Extend your left leg forward. Return to position 1. Repeat 8 times. Repeat 8 more times with your right leg. Continue for 3 sets of 8 extensions each, alternating left and right sides.

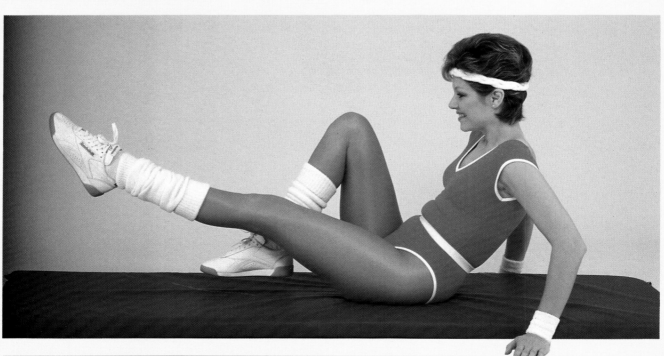

# WING IT

**1**

Sit erect, with the soles of your feet together and your knees bent to the sides as flat as possible. Hands are clasped behind the head.

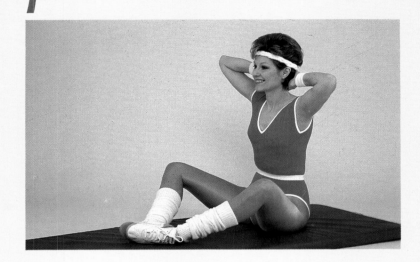

**2** Turn and touch your left elbow to the right knee. Return to position 1. Repeat, touching your right elbow to the left knee. Repeat, alternating left and right, 8 times. Continue for 3 sets of 8 each.

*This is a marvelous exercise for the waistline.*

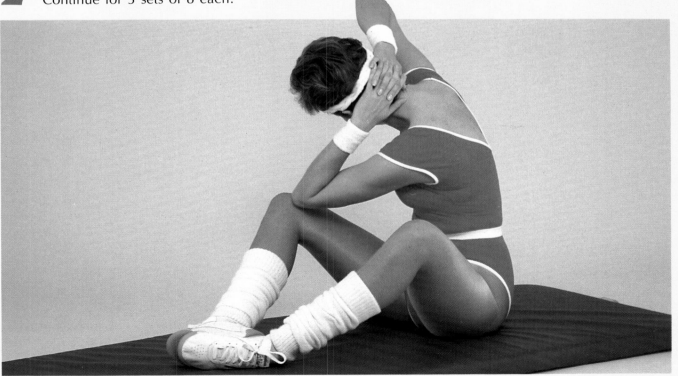

# SLIM THE SADDLEBAGS

## Day 4

**1**

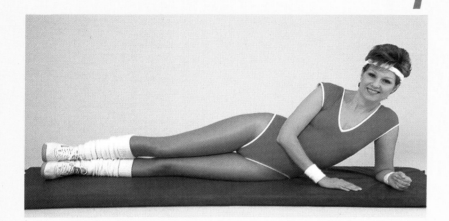

Lie on your left side with your legs extended, the right on top of the left. Your weight is on your left elbow. Use your right hand to support your body at the chest.

*Perfect for waist and hip "bags and sags"!*

Raise both legs as high as possible. (Don't expect to lift them too high.) Lower your legs and repeat 8 times. Switch sides and repeat. Continue for 3 sets of 8 times each, alternating sides after every 8 lifts.

**2**

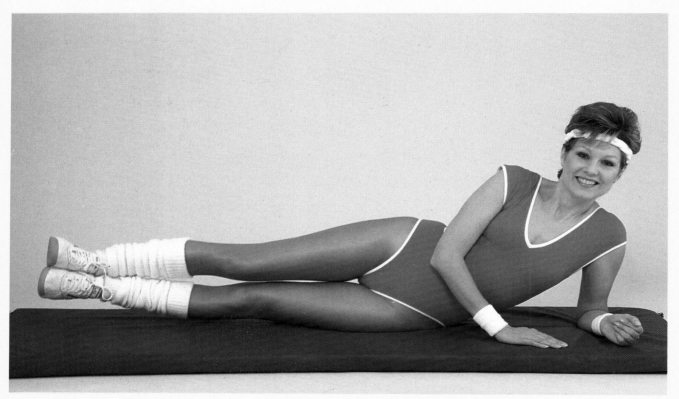

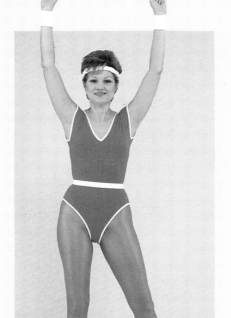

**1**

**2**

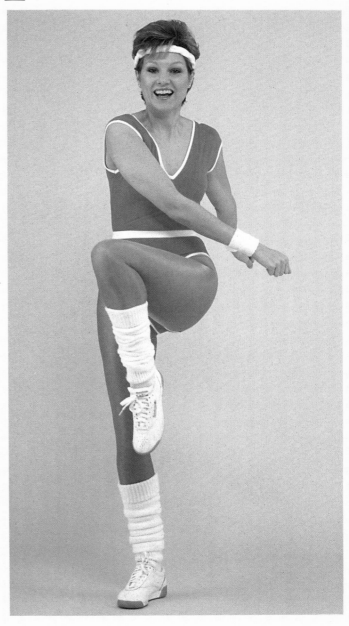

Stand with your feet slightly apart, weight on your right foot and left toe. Both arms are extended upward. Hands are held in fists—for power.

Raise your left knee and direct it across the body to the right. Lower both arms downward to the left side and directly toward the left hip. Do this forcefully—to burn lots of calories. Return to position 1. Repeat, 8 times left, 8 times right. Continue for 3 sets of 8 each, alternating sides.

*At this point you are ready for more difficult work.*

# MOVING UP

**1**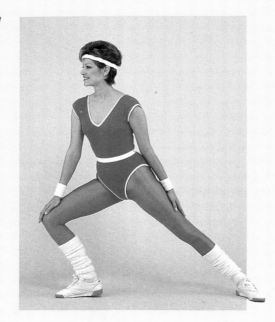

Stand with your feet wide apart. The right knee is bent, and the right toe is turned outward. The left leg is straight, with the left toe pointed forward. Place your right hand on your right knee for support; the left arm is at your side.

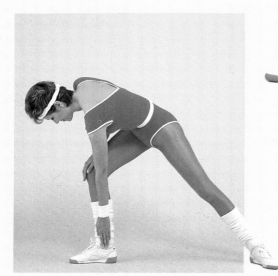

**2** Touch your right foot with your left hand.

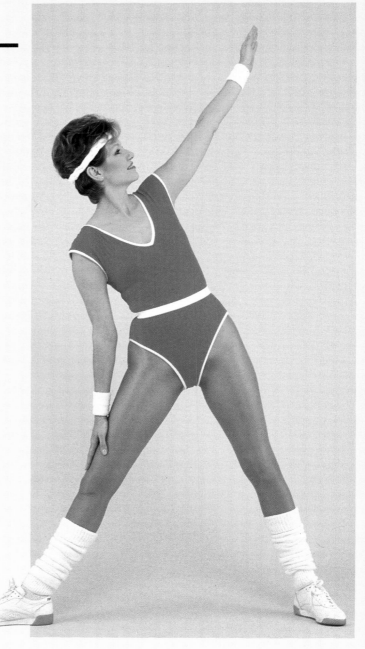

**3** Turning your torso and head toward the left arm, bring the left arm up and backward as far as possible. At the same time, straighten the right knee. Return to position 1 and repeat 8 times. Switch sides and repeat 8 more times. Continue for 3 sets of 8 each, alternating sides every 8 stretches.

*This is a strong lateral stretch—do it smoothly. Do not jerk or twist.*

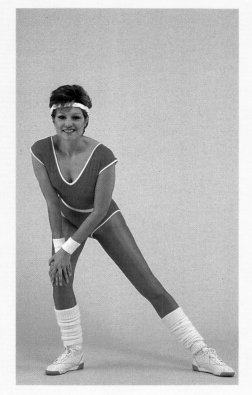

Stand with your feet wide apart. Facing forward, with both hands on your right knee, bend the right knee, and extend your left leg straight to the side. Your weight should be on your right foot and left toe.

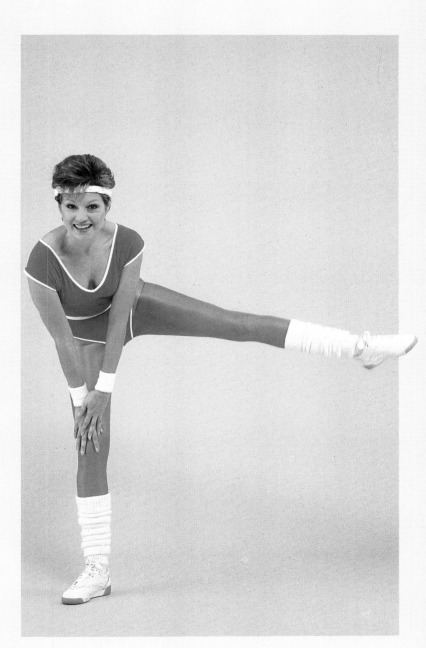

**2** Keeping your left leg DIRECTLY out to the side, raise it as high as possible. (Don't expect to lift it too high at first.) At the same time, straighten your right knee. Return to position 1. Repeat, 8 times left; 8 times right. Continue for 3 sets of 8 each, alternating sides.

*Great for waistline bulge.*

# DOUBLE DUTY

## Day 5

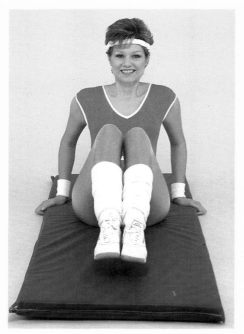

**1**

Sit with your weight on your hands, knees bent, and feet off the floor. Hunch your shoulders and round your back slightly (to prevent injury to the back).

**3** Return to position 1; extend both legs to the left side. Return to position 1; then extend both legs to the right side. Alternate left and right 8 times. Continue, alternating right and left for 3 sets of 8 each.

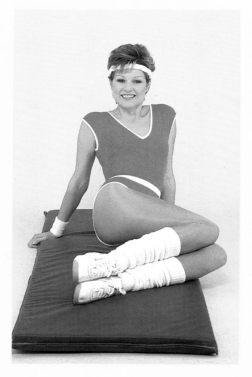

**2** Drop both knees to the left side, then to the right, alternating left and right 8 times. Continue the movement smoothly for 3 sets of 8 each. If you feel there is too much strain on your back, do this exercise while resting on your elbows.

**1**

Lie on your back with your head resting on the floor. Extend your left leg straight forward on the floor and right leg straight up. Extend your arms out to the sides.

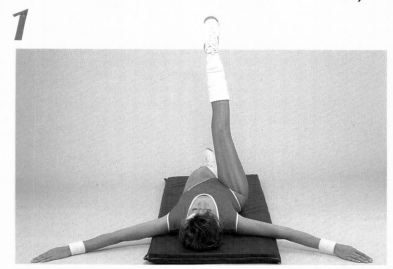

**2** Rolling on your left hip, lower your right leg, trying to touch your left hand. Return to position 1 and repeat 8 times. Reverse positions and repeat 8 times with the left leg and right hand. Continue for a total of 3 sets of 8 each, alternating sides after every 8 stretches.

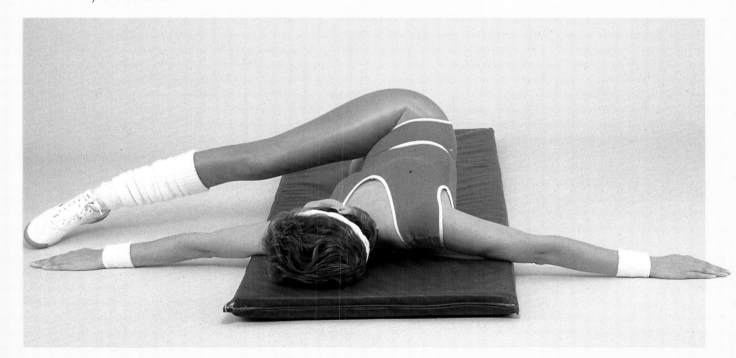

# SCISSOR STRETCH

*Day 5*

**1**

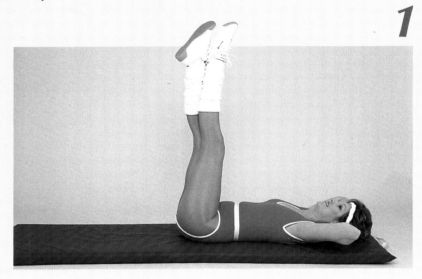

Lie on your back, legs extended upward, with your feet crossed at the ankles. Grasp your hands behind your head (your head may either be held up or resting on the floor, whichever is more comfortable for your back).

Lower both legs until you feel the pull in your abdominal muscles. Hold for 5 counts. Return to position 1. Repeat 8 times ONLY.

**2**

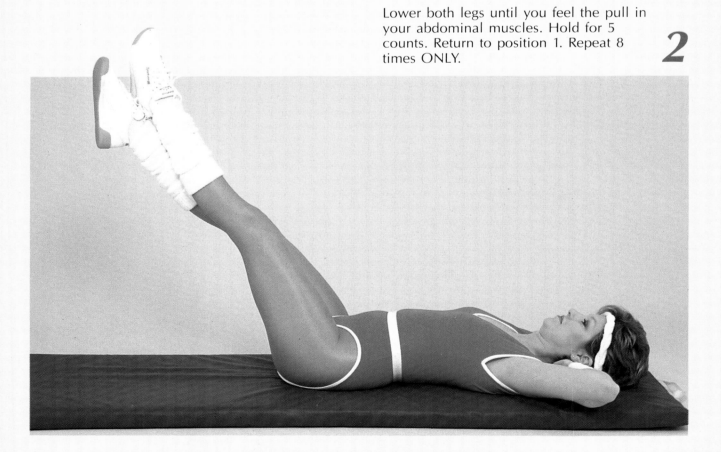

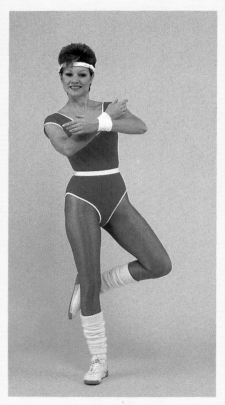

# FLY OUT

## DAY 6

**1** Stand erect with your weight on the right foot. Bend your left foot up behind the right. Cross your arms in front of your chest.

**2** Lunge to the left as far as possible. At the same time, extend your arms to the sides. Smoothly return to position 1. Repeat 8 times. Repeat 8 times to the right. Continue for 3 sets of 8, alternating sides.

*Do this exercise in a dance-type movement to assure maximum results—another great calorie burner.*

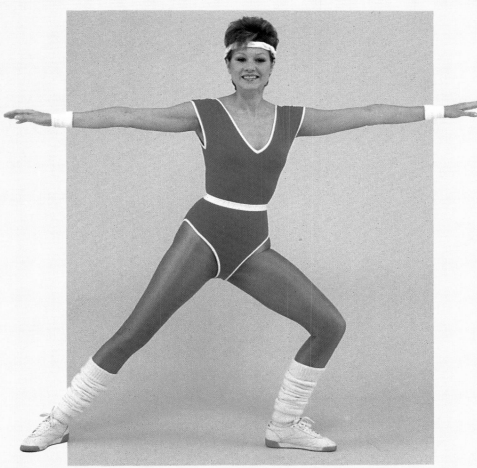

# ADVANCING

## Day 6

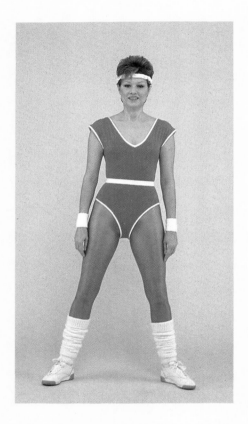

Stand erect with the feet wide apart, knees *slightly* bent. Arms are held at the sides.

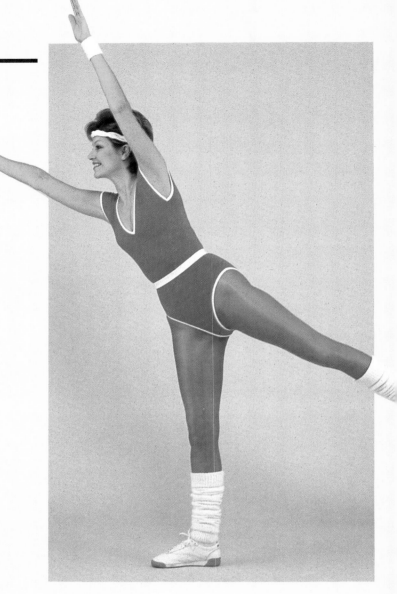

**2** Swing both arms up and across to the right. At the same time, raise the left leg as high as possible. Return to position 1. Swing both arms to the left, raising the right leg. Do this exercise in a continuous dance movement, alternating left and right for 3 sets of 8 swings.

# LOSE THE LUMPS

**1**

Sitting with your weight on your hands, shoulders hunched, back rounded, extend your legs upward.

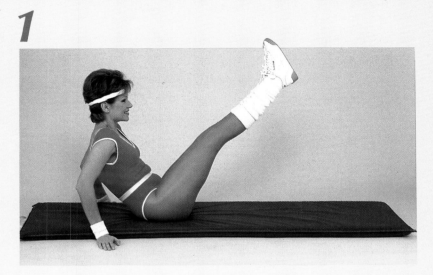

**2** Rotating on your hips and keeping your legs together, lower both legs to the right side. Return to position 1. Lower both legs to the left. Alternate right and left, 8 times. Continue for 3 sets of 8 stretches.

*If this exercise is too uncomfortable for your back, try doing it while resting on your elbows.*

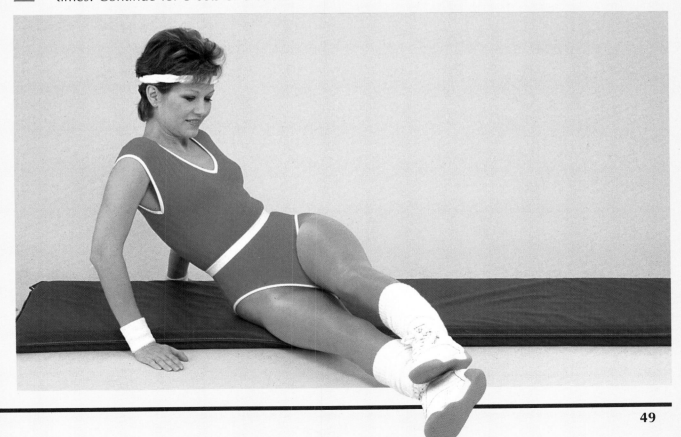

# FOR GREAT STATISTICS

*Day 6*

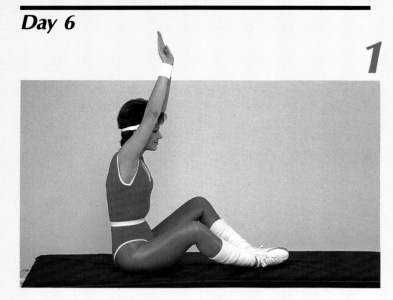

**1**

Sit erect with the soles of your feet together, knees bent to the sides. The arms are extended straight up, with the thumbs clasped.

Collapse (curl) your torso, rounding the back and tilting your pelvis upward. As you collapse, exhale. Inhale as you return to position 1. Repeat 8 times. Continue for 3 sets of 8 curls each.

*This is a complete abdominal exercise that also helps strengthen the back.*

**2**

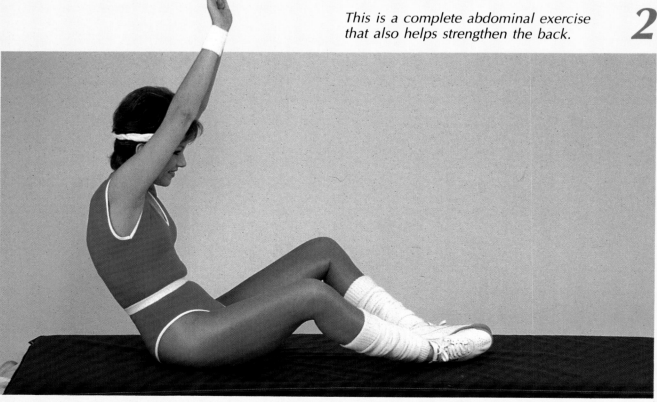

# CONTRACT THE MUSCLES

**1** Sit with the soles of your feet together, knees bent to the sides, weight on your elbows.

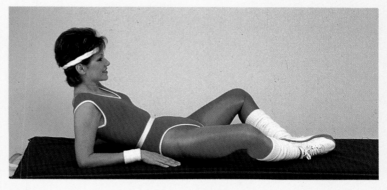

**2** Lift your elbows from the floor and slowly sit up and reach forward.

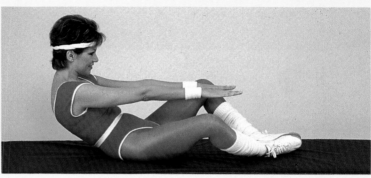

**3**

Reach as far forward as possible. Return to position 1 and repeat 8 times. Continue for 3 sets of 8 reaches.

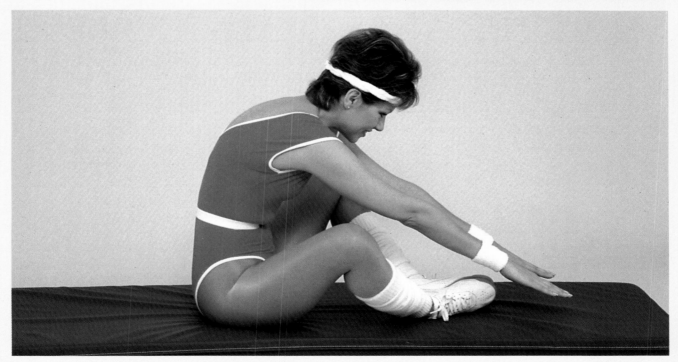

# SMOOTH OPERATION

## Day 6

**1**

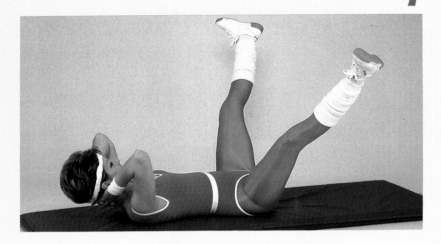

Lie on your back with your head up or resting on the floor (whichever is more comfortable), your hands clasped behind your head. Extend both legs upward and apart.

**2** Cross your legs, then open them—in a scissors motion. Continue "scissoring" while slowly lowering your legs halfway to the floor, then back up again. Continue to scissor for 4 counts up, 4 counts down. Repeat for 3 cycles of up and down scissoring.

*You should feel a long pull on the stomach muscles as you do this exercise.*

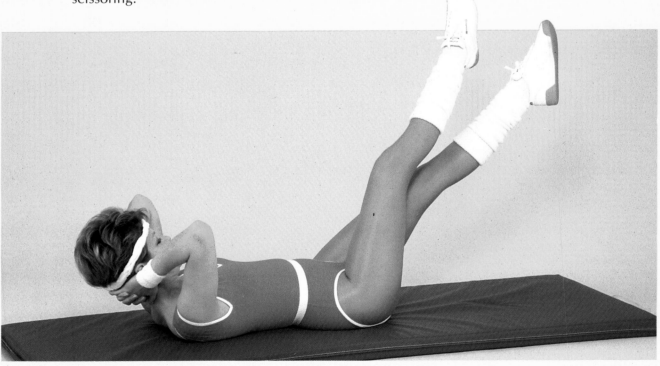

**1**

Lie on your back with your head and shoulders off the floor, chin on your chest, hands grasping the back of your thighs.

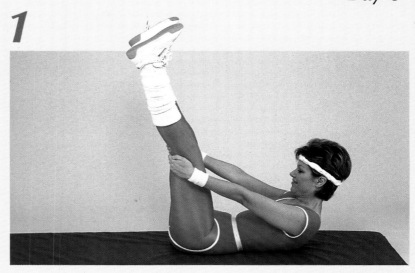

**2** Tightly grasp your thighs and raise your head and shoulders as high as possible. Try to keep your knees straight. Return to position 1. Repeat for 3 sets of 8 lifts each.

*Try to keep your legs in the starting position—try not to lower or "rock" them.*

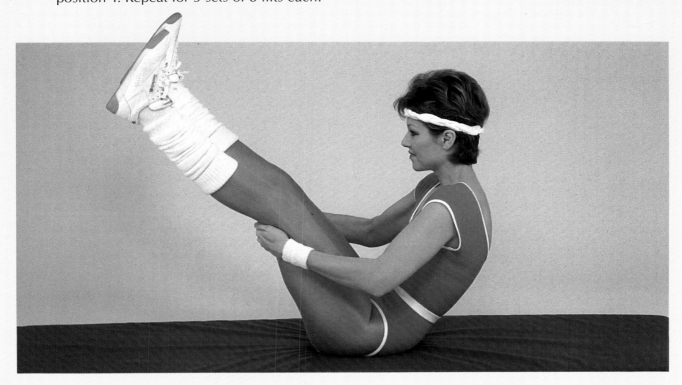

# CONTINUOUS FLOW

## DAY 7

**1**

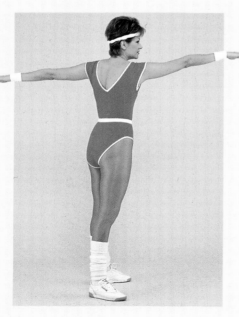

Stand erect with your feet wide
apart, head facing forward,
arms extended out to the sides.

**2** Rotate the right arm directly
forward, the left arm backward.

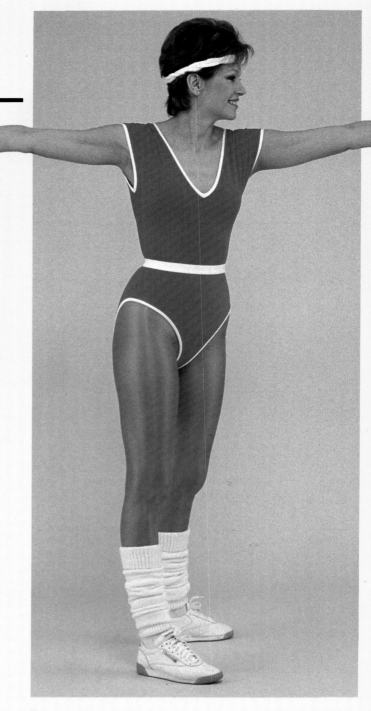

**3** Rotate your left arm forward and right arm
backward. Alternate for a total of 100
counts. Do this exercise quickly but
smoothly—do not stop between swings.

*For maximum firming of the abdominal
muscles without stressing the back, it is
important that you do not turn your head.*

**1**

Lie on your back with your head and shoulders off the floor, chin on your chest. The legs are wide apart with both feet flat on the floor. Place your hands at your sides, palms down on the floor.

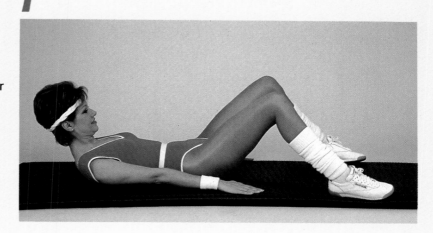

Raise your head and torso to a sitting position by sliding your hands along the floor toward your heels. Do not bend your elbows. Return to position 1—curl down smoothly. Repeat, for a total of 35 sits in one minute. Do not jerk your head.

*Guaranteed results!*

**2**

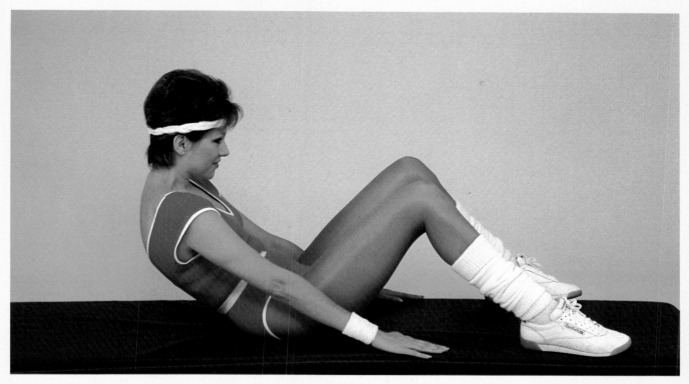

# POSITIVE ACTION

**Day 7**

**1**

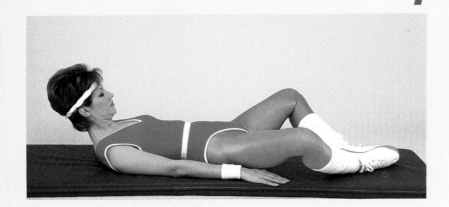

Lie on your back with your head and shoulders off the floor, chin on your chest, soles of your feet are flat together. Place your hands at your sides, palms down on the floor.

Lift your head and shoulders off the floor until you feel the contraction in your abdominal muscles. At the same time, slide your hands forward and exhale. Inhale as you return to position 1. Repeat for 3 sets of 8 sits.

**2**

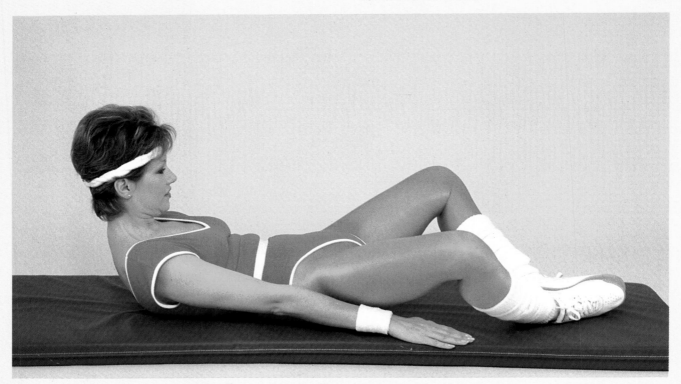

**1**

Sit with your left leg extended forward, right knee bent upward, right foot on the floor. Place your hands on either side of your right foot.

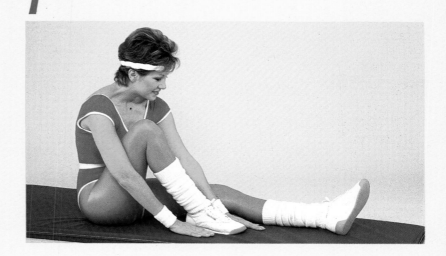

**2**

Keeping your hands on the floor next to your right foot, raise the left leg as high as possible. Hold for 5 counts. Lower, repeat 8 times. Repeat with right leg extended, left knee bent. Continue for 3 sets of 8 each, alternating left and right.

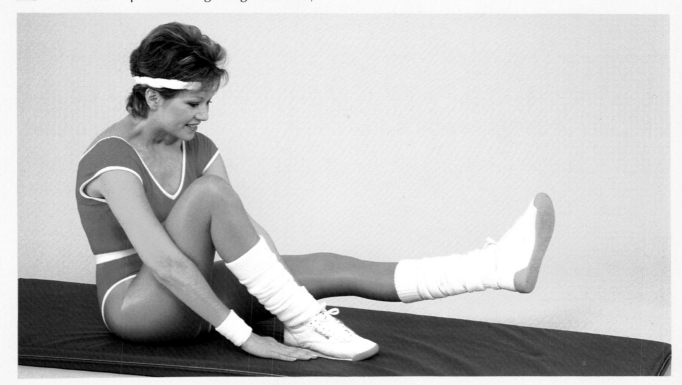

# MAXIMUM EFFORT

**Day 7**

**1**

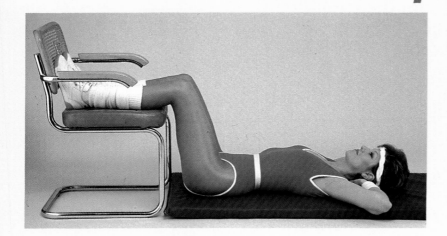

Lie on your back with your knees bent, calves on a chair, bed, or box (make sure it is very stable). Hold your hands behind your head, and scoot your hips toward the chair.

Lift your head and shoulders. Bring your elbows toward each other and try to touch your knees (or at least aim in that direction). Uncurl. Repeat 8 times ONLY.

*This is a very difficult exercise; do the best you can.*

**2**

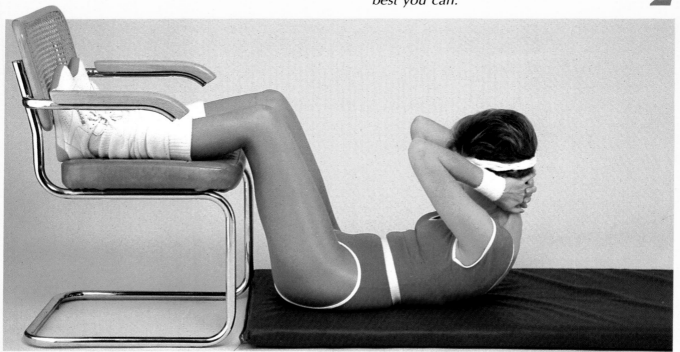

**1** Lie on your back with both knees bent toward the chest. Extend your arms sideways from the shoulders, hands touching the floor.

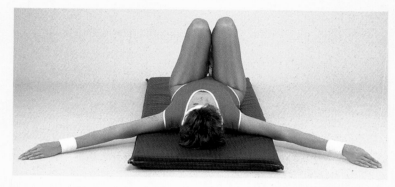

**2** Rotate your hips to the right side.

**3**

Extend your legs straight out. Return to position 1. Rotate your hips to the left, then extend your legs to the left. Alternate right and left 8 times. Continue for a total of 3 sets of 8 each.

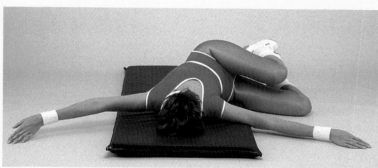

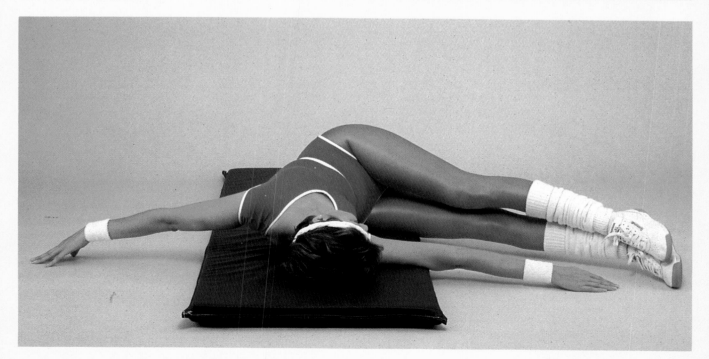

# FINAL ENTRY

## Day 7

**1**

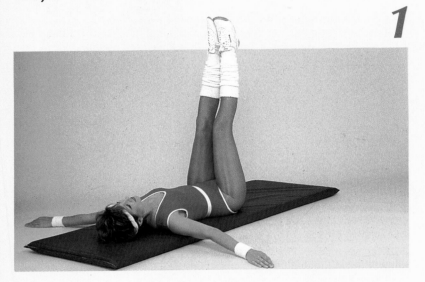

Lie on your back with both legs extended straight up. Extend your arms sideways from the shoulders.

Lower both legs to the right side, as close to your right hand as possible. Swing your legs up, then lower them to the left. Alternate right and left for 8 times ONLY.

*If you are very strong, continue for 3 sets of 8 swings.*

**2**

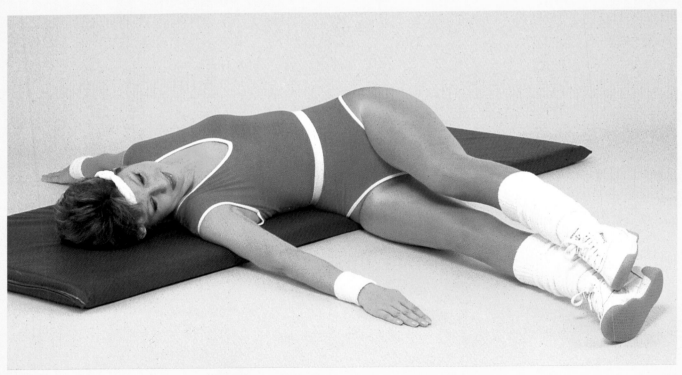

**1** Lie on your back with your head resting on the floor, hands behind your head. Knees are bent in toward your chest.

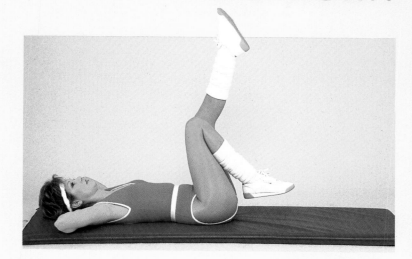

**2** Kick your legs up for 5 counts.

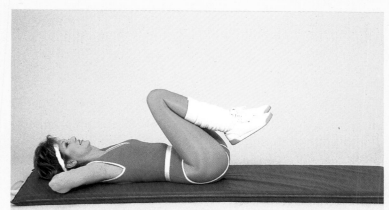

**3**

Kick your legs straight out for 5 counts. Repeat 5 times, alternately kicking up and straight out for a total of 50 kicks.

*Do this exercise lightly—without too much effort.*

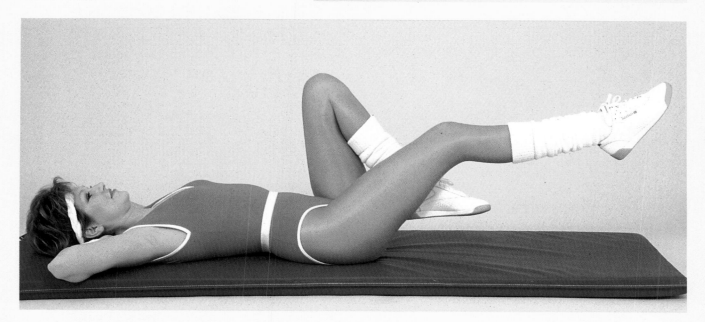

# OVERTIME REACH

## Cool Down

**1**

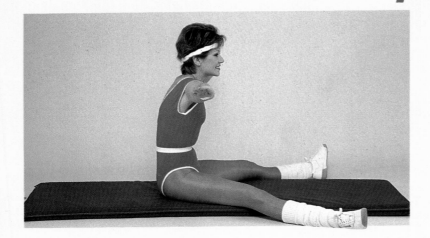

Sit erect on the floor with your legs wide apart, toes up. Extend your arms to the sides.

*A real plus for the back as well as the abdomen.*

Swing your left arm to touch your right toe. At the same time bring the right arm backward. Return to position 1. Swing your right arm to touch your left toe, bringing your left arm backward. Return to position 1. Continue, alternating right and left for a total of 50 swings.

**2**

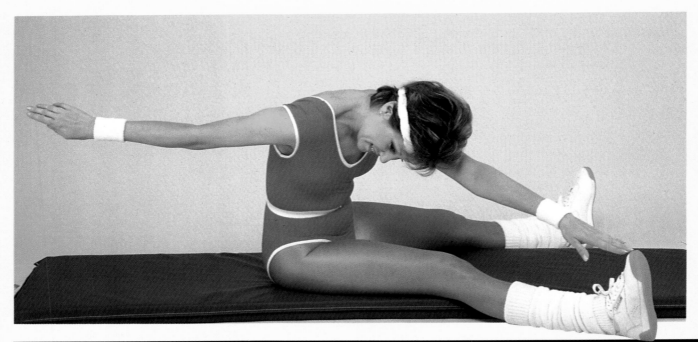

**1**

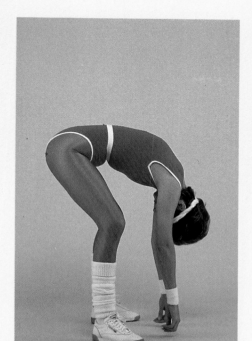

Stand with your feet apart, knees bent, your torso "collapsed," arms dangling toward the floor, your body relaxed.

**2**

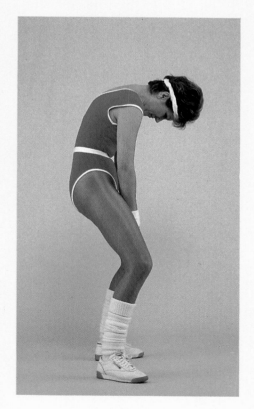

S-l-o-w-l-y uncurl.

# UNWIND
## *Cool Down*

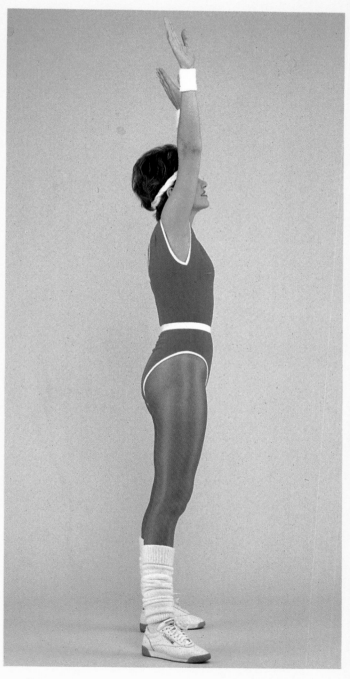

**3** Stretch your arms up toward the ceiling. Return to position 1. Repeat 3 times.

# TILT

## Cool Down

**1**

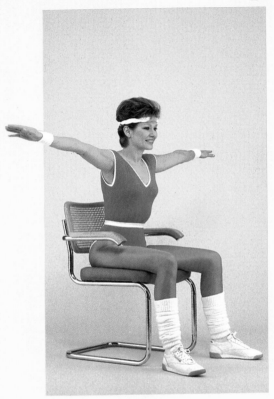

Sit erect in a sturdy chair, with both feet flat on the floor, legs wide apart. The back and hips are slightly away from the back of the chair. Extend your arms to the sides.

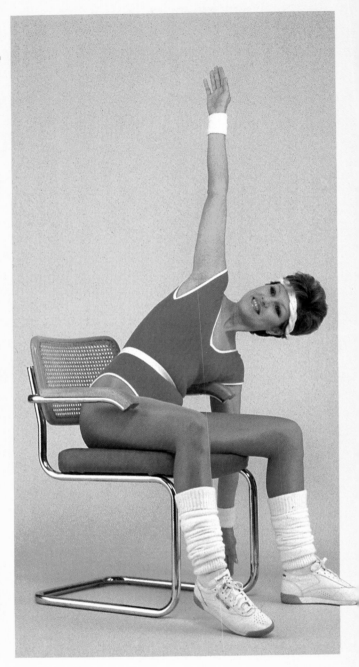

**2** Bend to the left and try to touch the floor with your left hand. (If you cannot reach the floor, don't try to reach any farther than you are able.) Extend your right hand straight up overhead. Repeat on the other side, with your right hand, and bending to the right. Repeat for 3 sets of 8 bends, alternating sides.

*This exercise is marvelous for the waistline.*